THE BEGINNER'S GUIDE TO STARTING GYM WORKOUTS

Description

Are you ready to take the first steps toward becoming a healthier, stronger, and more confident version of yourself? "The Beginner's Guide to Starting Gym Workouts" is your indispensable companion on the thrilling path to reaching your fitness objectives.

This thorough book is designed for those who are new to the world of gym routines, providing a clear and simple road map to success. Whether you want to lose weight, gain lean muscle, raise your energy, or simply improve your general well-being, this book will help you get there.

Learn how to develop attainable fitness goals based on your needs and objectives, giving you a clear sense of direction and motivation.

Learn how to use the most common gym equipment, such as treadmills and dumbbells, as well as weight machines, so you can easily navigate the gym floor.

Whether you're a complete beginner or have tried and failed in the past, this book will equip you with the knowledge, confidence, and motivation you need to embark on a successful fitness journey. Say goodbye to doubt and welcome to a healthier, happier self. Prepare to change your life one workout at a time. Begin reading "The Beginner's Guide to Starting Gym Workouts" right away!

TABLE OF CONTENTS

INTRODUCTION

IMPORTANCE OF REGULAR EXERCISE

Regular physical exercise is critical for general health maintenance. It is critical in supporting physical, mental, and emotional well-being. Regular exercise has several advantages that lead to a healthier and more enjoyable life.

First and foremost, regular exercise is essential for keeping a healthy body weight. Obesity is a major health problem worldwide, having far-reaching implications for an individual's well-being. Regular physical exercise aids in weight management by burning calories, building muscle, and improving metabolism. It also lowers the risk of obesity-related disorders, including type 2 diabetes and heart disease.

Exercise is essential for cardiovascular health in addition to weight management. It helps to strengthen the heart and improve circulation, lowering the risk of heart disease and stroke. Physical exercise helps lower blood pressure, lessen harmful cholesterol levels, and promote blood vessel health. These characteristics, taken together, lead to a healthy heart and a lower risk of cardiovascular disease.

Exercise is also important for preserving bone health and muscular strength. Bone density declines with age, leading to disorders such as osteoporosis. Walking, running, and weightlifting are all weight-bearing workouts that help stimulate bone development and preserve bone density. Likewise, muscle-strengthening exercises such as resistance training prevent age-related muscle loss while improving general physical strength and endurance.

In addition, regular exercise has a significant influence on mental health. It has been demonstrated to alleviate anxiety and depression symptoms, promote better sleep, and improve overall mood. Physical exercise causes the production of endorphins, sometimes known as "feel-good" chemicals, which contribute to a sense of well-being and stress reduction. Regular exercise regimens can also enhance cognitive function and memory, which is especially crucial as people age.

Exercise also has an important role in lowering the risk of chronic illnesses. Physical exercise has been associated with a lower risk of various illnesses, including breast and colon cancer. It also helps manage blood sugar levels, making it useful for people who have or are at risk of developing type 2 diabetes. Furthermore, exercise helps maintain a healthy immune system, making the body more capable of fighting infections and diseases.

Regular exercise promotes social contact and community participation in addition to physical advantages. Participating in group fitness classes, sports teams, or leisure activities in a nearby park can help foster social relationships and alleviate feelings of isolation. The sensation of belonging and camaraderie that frequently accompany group activities might benefit an individual's mental and emotional health.

Exercise is an important component in the context of lifespan. According to studies, individuals who engage in regular physical exercise live longer and have a superior quality of life in their older years. Staying active throughout life is essential for maintaining mobility, independence, and general health as one matures.

It is critical to underline that the advantages of regular exercise are not restricted to any one age group or fitness level. Everyone may benefit from adopting regular physical exercise into their daily routine, regardless of age, gender, or physical condition. Exercise may be adapted to individual interests and skills, ensuring everyone can find an appropriate approach to keeping active and healthy.

What type of Exercise is Right

Your fitness level, age, area of interest, health concerns, or impairments may influence the most beneficial physical activity. Walking, yoga, and cycling are low-impact exercises you may try while beginning your fitness routine. You could also exercise for shorter amounts of time.

According to the significance of physical activities on the EIT Food website, EIT Food suggests that children and adolescents should engage in around sixty minutes per day of moderate to intense activity, mostly aerobic. They should also engage in exercises that build their muscles and bones on three out of those seven days each week.

According to their findings, adults and older individuals should engage in 75-150 minutes of strenuous aerobic activity each week and 150-300 minutes of moderate aerobic activity. In addition to that, kids should engage in exercises that develop their muscles at least twice a week.

Let's go more into the primary and secondary forms of exercise that you should be doing. No matter what your current level of fitness is, Harvard University suggests that you engage in a variety of the following four primary forms of physical activity:

The Practice of Aerobics

Aerobic exercise is the same as cardiovascular exercise in that it speeds up your breathing and heart rate. It contributes to maintaining healthy blood vessels, heart, and lungs. Examples of this would be things like jogging, swimming, and doing Zumba, but it could also include things like playing football or tennis.

Workouts that Build Muscle

You will use equipment like dumbbells or your body weight in conjunction with resistance training to do this. Reducing the amount of fat in your body, preserving your muscle mass, and enhancing your bone health make you feel stronger and healthier.

An excellent illustration of this would be lifting weights.

To Stretch Out

This is the process of stretching or contracting particular muscles to increase the suppleness of those muscles. This results in improved flexibility, which leads to fewer injuries, improved posture, and relief from stress. There is a wide variety of exercises that focus on stretching, but in general, you will find that lessons in ballet or gymnastics contain a significant amount of stretching.

Harmony, Equilibrium

It doesn't matter if you're standing still or moving about; this test will determine how well you can retain your stance and keep your center of gravity in check. If you improve your balance, you will notice improvements in your posture, coordination, and the stability of your joints.

Maintaining your balance becomes increasingly crucial as you become older because of the increased risk of falling. Various activities might help you improve your balance, but gymnastics and surfing are two examples of sports that need balance.

BENEFITS OF EXERCISE

Because there are so many benefits to exercise and physical activity, we'll give you a quick review of the key ones before getting into more depth on illness prevention and mental health. These are some examples:

- Bones, muscles, and joints that are stronger
- Weight loss, muscle gain, and fat loss
- Skin improvement
- Reduce your blood pressure
- Inflammation is reduced.
- Stress levels have been reduced.
- Enhanced mood
- increased clarity of thought
- Immune system boost Improved cognitive function
- Fewer injuries from falls

THE ROLE OF EXERCISE IN DISEASE PREVENTION

Adults who participate in regular physical activity and exercise have a lower risk of death from various diseases and conditions, including cardiovascular disease, cancer, type 2 diabetes, and others. One of the primary reasons for this is due to the fact that physical activity has an anti-inflammatory impact.

Inactivity raises the risk of obesity as well as the diseases that were discussed before. This is due to the fact that having a significant level of body fat can lead to inflammation. When muscles are worked out, chemicals, including adrenaline, cortisol, and the cytokine IL-6, are released into the bloodstream. Exercise has been shown to have anti-inflammatory benefits, and as a result, regular exercise can reduce the risk of illness brought on by inflammation.

CHAPTER 1: GETTING STARTED

MENTAL PREPARATION

Before you go onto a treadmill or pick up a weight, consider three important aspects of fitness: motivation, humility, and objectives.

Motivation

Ask yourself why you're doing this. Is it only for you? Your partner? What about your kids? It may be for a buddy who is overweight and needs a little push to start working out. Whether a single element or a combination of factors, the urge to be in shape will be the driving force behind every workout.

There will be moments when you want to avoid working out when you first start or are six months into a fitness regimen. You just will not. It would be best to remind yourself why you're working out on these occasions. Other apocalyptic scenarios inspire you to exercise, but I won't explore them here. Instead, consider some nicer, more appropriate reasons.

Perhaps you're sick of standing on the porch watching your kids play football in the backyard and want to join them. Perhaps you'd want to be more than a puffing and wheezing blob to your partner in an intimate scenario. It might be as basic as wanting to remove your shirt at the beach without feeling self-conscious. You don't have to have six-pack abs, but you should feel good about yourself.

When you've determined why you want to get back in shape, find a means to remind yourself of it. I was never a fan of writing inspiring messages on your bathroom mirror or wearing a bracelet with an inspirational message on it. It would be best to be reminded of your motivation rather than suffocated by it. I have a high school snapshot of me taken the day before my final year of basketball practice. After a full-contact football game, several buddies and I snapped a silly snapshot standing with our shirts off. That was the greatest shape I'd ever been in. I'd look at the photo to remind myself that I could have a high fitness level. It's up to you how you remind yourself, but make sure you do it.

Humility

YOU ARE NO LONGER 17 YEARS OLD. Got it? When people ask me how to return to the gym, I tell them that the first time isn't the most difficult; it's the second time many guys fail. Too often, guys fail in their fitness goals because they act like they're still 17 and go full speed on the first session. If you don't pull a hammy during the exercise, you'll feel like you went three rounds with Kimbo Slice the next morning. You can hardly stand because your knees, back, and neck suffer. So, when you think of your next workout, the words 'Hell' and 'No' normally come to mind.

I'll go into a strategy in later columns, but here's how I began with my exercises last spring: 30 minutes of walking at 2.4 miles per hour with varied degrees of inclination on the treadmill. It's tough to appear cool when slogging away on a treadmill, pouring with sweat. On the other hand, starting slowly will create a firmer basis for fitness development. Getting over the ego component of 'looking cool' while working out necessitates humility.

Goals

Setting and achieving goals is an important component of getting back in shape. Having a goal to strive towards as a measure of achievement gives positive reinforcement that your efforts are worthwhile. The bathroom scale is the most straightforward aim to establish. Choose a number to read and proceed to that number. It would be best if you talked to your doctor about this. Goals might be minor or enormous in scale. You may only wish to run a mile without stopping, lose 10 pounds, or finish a 5K event.

The best part about your objectives is that you can quickly make new ones once you've completed the others. My initial objective was to complete a 10K run. I reasoned that if I could achieve that, everything else - reducing weight, stopping smoking, getting in shape - would fall into place. That's exactly what occurred in September when I ran a 10K.

But don't set too lofty a goal; you want to achieve it in a fair length of time. You may aspire to run a marathon someday, but a 2-mile fun run may be a great place to start. The important thing to remember is that getting back into shape is achievable no matter how out of shape you believe you are. It took you years to get to this position, but you can return on track in a few weeks. You'll be a better man as a result of it.

IMPORTANCE OF SETTING CLEAR FITNESS GOALS

Goal setting is a mental training strategy determining specified, measurable, and time-bound objectives. Does that make sense? We often establish hundreds upon hundreds of objectives for ourselves every day without even realizing it. These can range from picking up milk at the corner store, making toast, or simply setting the alarm clock or changing the channel on the television (short-term goals) to graduating from university, becoming a millionaire within the next ten to fifteen years, or saving for a once-in-a-lifetime trip around the world (long term goals). Goal setting is something you must rely on to live regularly as a human being. Goal setting, on the other hand, is not only an essential component of successful everyday life; it is also a proven strategy (and hence an indispensable component) of effective sporting performance, adopted by practically all sports performers worldwide!

Goals have been shown to boost performance levels by 16% on average. The incorporation of goal setting into your training regimen may have four significant effects on your performance:

1. GOALS GIVE GUIDANCE

They guide your training by directing your attention away from goal-irrelevant activities and toward goal-relevant ones. If a marathon runner wants to enhance his cardiovascular fitness, running economy, and muscular strength, he should concentrate on these areas (goal-relevant activities). Other duties should not be prioritized, such as strengthening his throwing capacity or free-throw ability (goal-irrelevant activities). This strategy would allow him to concentrate on the most critical areas of his training, ensuring that it is as efficient and successful as possible.

2. GOALS MOTIVATE PEOPLE

Goals enable you to easily analyze performance and learn more about your training skills, which may then assist in replacing monotony with the challenge, i.e., goals function as an energizer! You will develop self-directed motivation as you achieve your objectives, replacing anxiety and stress with focus and confidence. These variables, when combined, frequently result in more gratifying training.

For example, an overweight guy attempting to drop 50 pounds may regard this as impossible, especially given that he has been overweight for much of his life. However, by setting a target of losing two pounds each week and tracking his progress, he may stay motivated and stay on track (persist) with the weight reduction program until the end goal is reached. Similarly, a middle-distance runner who wants to cut five minutes off her 10 km race time may not want to put in the necessary mileage day after day. Setting short-term targets, such as lowering her run time by 5-10 seconds each day, helps her to see her progress toward her long-term goal on a daily basis, giving her training a daily purpose while also allowing motivation to be maintained on a daily and long-term basis.

3. GOALS ENABLE THE ESTABLISHMENT OF APPROPRIATE LEARNING TECHNIQUES

When goals are established, the person and coach may create and implement methods to achieve the individual's short and long-term sports objectives. Suppose a novice swimmer wants to improve their core stability. In that case, they (the individual and coach/personal trainer) may perform two to three core exercises at the end of every other gym workout or change their core exercise technique to make their routine more efficient and effective.

So far, we have spoken about how important goal setting is for exercise, but to get the most out of it, there are a few things you need to think about beforehand. We go into more detail about this in our 'How to Remain Focused on Your Gym Goals' post, but for now, let us focus on the fact that there are three unique sorts of goals (outlined below). The crucial element to remember here is that you should ideally mention each objective during goal planning. Your attention should not be just on obtaining your ultimate goal (which is sometimes so simple to do).

(1) Process Objectives

This entails completing a task and improving your skill level. You have total control over your process goals, which may be quite helpful in lowering anxiety before an event. Here are several examples:

• Improving your diet • Performing a pre-performance ritual, such as self-talk or listening to your favorite music on your MP3 player • Getting adequate sleep and relaxation to promote recovery • Sticking to your training plan as strictly as possible; • communicating with your instructor on a regular basis; and • keeping your equipment in good condition.

(2) Performance Objectives

Performance objectives establish a precise benchmark to be met (usually based on your expectations). These can range from losing a certain amount of weight in a given time to jogging a certain distance on a treadmill. Performance objectives are unaffected by the performance of others and are thus entirely within your control. They can make you happy even if you don't accomplish your objective.

(3) Outcome Objectives

These objectives relate to the final product or, to put it another way, the desired result, such as winning a race or defeating an opponent. These are extremely motivating objectives, but unlike process goals, they are not always under the individual's control. They are influenced by how others perform and how successfully you apply your process and performance targets.

Setting goals is an exceptionally effective method for improving performance, and it is a strategy that can be utilized by almost anybody, from the most accomplished athletes to casual gym-goers. Your goals may assist you in determining your final location, provide you with a practical means of determining the paths you can follow to get there, and inform you when you have arrived at your objective. It is vital to evaluate the various kinds of goals and the ways in which they may be included in your training regimen so that you can keep your attention on the objectives you have set for the gym.

CHAPTER 2: CHOOSING THE RIGHT GYM

Whether you aim to lose weight, tone up, or live a better lifestyle, attending a gym will be an important part of your fitness journey. Because everyone has various requirements and desires when selecting a gym, you may limit your options depending on your fitness goals.

THINGS TO CONSIDER WHEN CHOOSING A GYM

1. Ease of use

If you want to avoid the possibility of finding reasons to skip an exercise, convenience is the most important thing to consider. You are significantly less likely to visit a gym if it is too far out of your way. If, on the other hand, your gym is close to home or on your way home from work, you'll find it easy to persuade yourself to go and put in the effort. You'll be able to spend more time exercising than driving to the gym since you won't have to factor in a long trip.

2. Tradition

Look for a gym with a warm, welcoming atmosphere. When you're in the gym and feel at ease, you're more likely to enjoy your workout, motivating you to keep going. Look for a member-focused club that suits your training style to locate the gym that will help you the most on your fitness quest.

Consider the gym's target demographic and whether you meet the profile. For those new to working out, a gym full of "bros" and bodybuilders might be scary, and they should seek out a less intensive facility. If your gym has outlawed grunting in the weight room and you have a habit of being rather noisy when lifting, you may want to seek a better match. 5 Bridges Health & Fitness works hard to establish a culture suitable for everyone, from beginners to fitness enthusiasts to elders.

3. Courses

The gym's group workout courses will be key to your membership experience. Whether you enjoy spinning, Zumba, kickboxing, yoga, barre, or another kind of exercise, be sure your gym provides group sessions at times that work for you. Find a gym that offers certified personal trainers in addition to group workout sessions. Working with a personal trainer is one of the greatest methods to reach your fitness objectives, so be sure your gym has certified trainers on staff who are eager to help you design a successful course and lead you through how to optimize your time at the gym. If you can find a personal trainer with whom you click, your fitness journey will be much easier.

4. Cleanliness

Gyms, a social space where everyone sweats, create the ideal habitat for germs to increase if not adequately cleaned. Take note of whether personnel wipe down the gym's equipment on a regular basis and whether members adhere to a tight cleanliness policy. Consider whether or not the gym supplies sanitizing wipes or a spray bottle with paper towels to sanitize equipment and whether or not people utilize them.

In addition to the gym, examine the toilets and locker rooms. If these locations aren't clean, the facility will probably do everything possible to sterilize and safeguard guests' health. In addition to basic hygiene, ensure that your chosen gym complies fully with state and municipal COVID-19 safety rules.

5. Overcrowding

A gym may contain every piece of workout equipment imaginable, but it is only useful if that equipment is available. Please stop by the gym you want to join when you're most likely to work out to observe how crowded it is. If there constantly seems to be a big queue for specific equipment, particularly ones you use most frequently, consider visiting another gym where you can spend more time working out and less time waiting in line.

6. Gym Hours

You only have so much time to spare between job, family, and (of course) sleep. As a result, a fitness club that opens late and shuts early is unlikely to suit your needs.

When looking into a gym, find out the hours and what is available throughout those hours. When will trainers be available? Are there any facilities or areas of the gym that are closed at specific times? It's critical to understand the club's hours and offers so you can organize your training routine properly.

7. Location Should be Optimized

Location, location, and location are all important. In addition to being vital for the success of a business, the location of your gym is of the utmost significance to the training regimen you follow. If you have to travel thirty minutes to get to your gym, you may likely skip more workouts than you complete. The amount of time you can devote to working out is also significantly impacted by the time it takes you to and from the gym. I've discovered that somewhere between five and fifteen minutes is the optimal time to drive to the gym. If it takes you any longer, getting to the gym will be easier than going to work.

8. Be Sure to Look out for any Additional Charges

"Join now for the low price of only $1!" Have you seen any of such advertisements on your travels? I do not doubt that. The majority of gyms use this method to entice customers to join —offerings with low barriers to entry that are almost too good to be true. A gym membership contract typically contains a significant amount of legalese. The majority of fitness centers charge their members an additional cost known as a maintenance and enhancement fee on top of their regular monthly dues. This fee is intended to "enhance" the fitness center. It would be best if you inquired about any costs that come along with maintaining your membership. Check to see what is included and what would be an additional cost. Before you put your name on the dotted line, be sure you get all of your questions answered.

9. You Can Test Before You Buy

Before you decide to acquire a gym membership, using the facility's free visitor pass is usually a good idea. Before making a long-term commitment to a gym, it is important to become familiar with all of the equipment, observe the surrounding area, and try out a variety of workout schedules. Working out at the facility for a week might give you a fair idea of whether or not you enjoy being there.

10. Feel Out the Atmosphere

Is the thought of entering the gym enough to motivate you to lift ridiculously heavy weights, or are you finding that the gym is putting you to sleep? It would be best if you inquired about the quality of the lifting atmosphere at the gym to ensure that it will meet your needs. Other gyms don't appear to have any "energy," and the environment is nearly completely lifeless. On the days that you don't feel like working out, this may not seem like a huge problem, but trust me, it is. You want to go into a setting that inspires you and gets your blood pumping as soon as you get there.

When searching for the ideal fitness center, it is important to take several important considerations into account, including the following: location, working hours, pricing, equipment, cleanliness, trainer credentials, environment, and cancellation policies. Spend time researching and going to several gyms to discover the facility that caters to your fitness needs and tastes. You can guarantee that you have a good and fruitful experience on your fitness journey by making decisions based on accurate information.

CHAPTER 3: UNDERSTANDING GYM EQUIPMENT

TYPES OF GYM EQUIPMENT COMMONLY FOUND IN FITNESS CENTERS

If you are still getting familiar with how to use them, the exercise equipment at the gym might be really scary. If you are still getting familiar with typical gym equipment and the muscles they train, it may be difficult to plan and carry out an efficient exercise using such machines.

To our good fortune, the majority of fitness centers offer comparable amenities. As soon as you are comfortable with the fundamental equipment in your location, you will be able to step into any gym confidently and immediately begin your exercise.

THE 5 MOST POPULAR CARDIO MACHINES

The majority of gyms have machines that can assist in increasing your aerobic fitness, cause you to burn calories, and enhance the health of your heart. These five mainstays are the most frequent types of cardiac exercise equipment used at the gym, even though the brands and styles may differ.

Elliptical Machine

Elliptical machines provide a smoother ride than treadmills, enabling users to replicate walking or running movements without impact. The elliptical footpad stays beneath your foot throughout each stride, so there is no impact during turnover. Some elliptical machines feature moving arm grips, while others have fixed rails.

You will step up onto the footpads before turning on an elliptical machine. Use the handrails for balance as you pick a pre-programmed workout or your favorite time and level. When the machine starts moving, the footpads guide your foot through each stride. If it feels too simple, up the difficulty level to make each stage more difficult.

STATIONARY BICYCLE

Stationary bikes at the gym give an indoor cycling experience. Traditional upright and recumbent bikes are available at most gyms. Many gyms offer spin bike-based indoor cycling group exercise courses. Each form of stationary bike may help you increase your cardiovascular fitness as well as build your lower body muscles (quadriceps, hamstrings, glutes, and calves).

Follow the directions on the machine to properly set the seat height and lead your first exercise, whether using a standard or recumbent stationary bike. Add enough resistance to make it feel like you're riding across soft terrain rather than spinning through thin air.

TREADMILL

A treadmill allows you to walk, jog, run, or mix these modes into an interval workout. Treadmills are gentler on the joints than running outside, and they allow you to manage the intensity of your workout so that you may attain a target heart rate to fulfill fitness objectives.

To operate a treadmill, first step upon the deck before turning on the machine. The treadmill deck is the stationary region that surrounds the belt. Set a leisurely walking speed by pressing the start button. Step onto the belt and begin walking. When you feel comfortable and stable, raise the tempo or incline to achieve the desired workout intensity.

Climber of Stairs

These "stairs to nowhere" provide a challenging aerobic exercise while strengthening the lower body. Some stair steppers include footpads that stay beneath your feet throughout each stride, comparable to an elliptical. On the other hand, other gym machines resemble an escalator and force you to elevate your foot with each step.

Begin by taking modest steps that do not require a large "lift" with each repeat while utilizing a stair stepper or climbing machine. Most machines offer a quick start button at the most basic level. As you increase your level, you'll find that each step grows steeper and more difficult.

Rower

Rowers simulate boat rowing, offering excellent aerobic exercise while strengthening the legs, chest, and back. Rowing machines are commonly used in boot camp-style exercises because they provide an effective total-body workout.

To begin using a rowing machine, sit on the molded seat and place your feet on the footpads. Tighten the straps to secure your feet, then hold the rowing handle overhand. Pull the grip towards your body while straightening your legs in a rowing action. Repeat the maneuver in the other direction.

5 WELL-KNOWN STRENGTH MACHINES

Most gyms include equipment to help you grow muscle and increase your strength. For example, in the free weight training section, you will likely encounter dumbbells, barbells with weight plates, and kettlebells.

However, there is always a section where you may locate strength training exercise machines. According to the International Sports Science Association (ISSA), machines are frequently safer in the beginning since they provide greater stability, albeit certain machines provide more stability than others.

These five popular gym strength training devices will help you obtain a full-body strength exercise. Read the directions on each machine carefully to discover how to remain safe and maximize each movement.

Press the Chest

The seated chest press machine works to build your pectoralis muscles at the front of your chest, your triceps muscles in the rear of your arm, and your deltoid or shoulder muscles.

To operate the machine, sit on a cushioned seat, press grips away from the torso to an extended position (with elbows practically straight), then bend at the elbow to control the release back toward the body.

Pulldown Lat

The lat pull targets the latissimus dorsi muscle, a big wing-shaped muscle in your mid-back. This machine has a seat as well as an interchangeable bar or grips that dangle over your head.

Grab the overhead bar or handles with your hands slightly wider than shoulder distance apart to do the lat pulldown. Pull the bar down towards your upper chest while seated, then return to the beginning position and repeat.

Leg Extensions

By situating your body such that your legs must lift weight away from your hips, the leg press machine helps you build the muscles in your lower body (glutes, hamstrings, and quadriceps).

Sit in the comfortable seat and set your feet on the broad platform to perform the leg press. Once you're in position (ankles and knees aligned with hips), bring the platform closer to your body so your knees are bent and near your chest. Different machines have various levers that aid in this action. Finally, press the platform away from your body using your leg muscles until your knees are fully stretched, then reverse and repeat.

The Smith Machine

The Smith machine can help a weighted squat workout by anchoring and directing the barbell's motions. Some people use a Smith machine for a chest press when reclining on a weight bench.

Start with the bar racked (no weight on your body) and place it such that it rests on the meaty region of your upper shoulders to do a squat exercise on a Smith machine. With an overhand grip, place your hands on the bar at shoulder height. Remove the bar from the rack by rotating it back slightly and lowering the hips into a deep squat position. Repeat the maneuver in the other direction. Before leaving the machine, complete the necessary repetitions and re-rack the weight.

Cables

This huge device is a multipurpose equipment with cables and pulleys for strength exercises. The amazing thing about this gym equipment is that it comes with various attachments, and most settings have detailed instructions.

Cables, for example, may be utilized to do biceps curls on the front of the upper arm, triceps extensions on the rear of the upper arm, and even aided pull-ups on the upper back and arms.

HOW TO USE MACHINES, FREE WEIGHTS, AND CARDIO EQUIPMENT

Gym equipment comes in various shapes and sizes, each with a unique training purpose. A balanced exercise plan requires a proper understanding of utilizing machines, free weights, and cardio equipment. Here's how to utilize each piece of equipment:

1. MECHANICAL DEVICES

Machines are intended to offer certain muscular areas with stability and isolation. They are appropriate for novices as well as those wishing to target certain regions of their body.

a. Choose the Right Machine: Select a machine that targets the muscle group you wish to focus on. Choose a leg press machine, for example, to train your quadriceps.

b. Change the Seat and Settings: The majority of machines offer adjustable chairs and weight stacks. Check that the seat is at the proper height and that the weight is appropriate for your fitness level.

c. Maintain good Form: To guarantee good form, follow the directions on the equipment or see a trainer. This lowers your chance of injury while increasing the efficacy of your workout.

d. Movement Control: Concentrate on controlled and purposeful motions across the whole range. When lifting the weight, avoid utilizing momentum.

e. Do Sets and Repetitions: Incorporate machines into your training program by doing a certain number of sets and repetitions for each activity.

2. BODYWEIGHT

Dumbbells and barbells, for example, demand more stability and work for several muscle groups, making them ideal for functional strength training.

a. Begin with a Warm-up: To prepare your muscles for the workout, begin with a warm-up. Light aerobic or dynamic stretching might be beneficial.

b. Choose the Appropriate Weight: Select weights that will challenge you while allowing you to retain good form. Begin with lesser weights and progressively increase as your strength increases.

b. Maintain Proper Form: Maintain proper form to avoid injury. Maintain core engagement, a full range of motion, and weight management throughout the exercise.

d. Include Compound Exercises: Free weights are ideal for compound exercises such as squats, deadlifts, and bench presses, which train numerous muscular groups at the same time.

b. Include Variety: To target different muscle groups and avoid plateaus, incorporate various free weight exercises within your regimen.

3. CARDIOVASCULAR EQUIPMENT

Treadmills, stationary cycles, and elliptical machines are cardio equipment used to enhance cardiovascular fitness, burn calories, and increase endurance.

a. Warm-up: Begin with a warm up session on the cardio equipment to gradually boost your heart rate. Walking or leisurely cycling can be used as warm-ups.

b. Determine Your Intensity: Change the resistance or pace to suit your fitness level and goals. Beginners might begin with lesser settings and progressively increase them.

b. Maintain appropriate Posture: Maintain appropriate posture to avoid strain or pain. Maintain a straight back and use your core muscles.

d. Interval Training: Include interval training between high and low-intensity intervals. This can increase calorie burn while also improving cardiovascular fitness.

g. Heart Rate Monitor: Some cardio equipment have heart rate monitors. Monitoring your heart rate might assist you in remaining in your desired training zone for the best outcomes.

f. Cool Down: Follow up your aerobic workout with a cool-down session in which you progressively reduce the intensity to allow your heart rate to return to normal.

SAFETY TIPS AND PROPER TECHNIQUES FOR USING GYM EQUIPMENT

Get a Health Checkup Every Year

Diabetes and heart disease may creep up on even the most active persons, so schedule your regular checkup. Most clubs and fitness programs may suggest or demand a checkup to verify you don't have a medical condition that particular forms of activity could exacerbate. However, you must remember to schedule the appointment every year.

Consult your doctor about your fitness goals, especially if you have a prior condition or are using drugs. Most doctors will support your desire to become more active. However, you may be offered limits or cautions if you have certain health concerns or dangers.

Perform a Warm-up and a Cool-down.

Warming up properly helps flow blood to your muscles and prepare you for additional exercise. Begin your cardio workout (treadmill, elliptical, or stationary cycle) at a leisurely pace and light intensity for three to five minutes before increasing your exertion to your desired level. After your primary activity, take a few minutes to cool down at a reduced level of intensity.

Warming up for strength training and other workout activities with three to five minutes of treadmill walking or walking in place can assist in getting the blood flowing to your muscles and help them perform better. Do stretching and mobility exercises before commencing any workout to prepare your body for the work ahead.

Gradually Increase the Amount

If you progressively increase an activity's time, intensity, or reps, your body will benefit greatly from the training impact. A terrific physique develops slowly, and doing too much too soon increases your risk of injury and consequences.3

In your workout training, use the correct progression:

Increase the duration and work on your technique before raising your speed and intensity level for cardiac activity. Start with smaller weights and gradually increase repetitions and sets before increasing weight. Every 4-6 weeks, re-evaluate your program and consider making changes.

Use Proper Technique

The manner in which you perform the exercise is vital for achieving good results and avoiding harm. If you lift weights in a way that stresses your lower back, you will experience discomfort. Aches, pains, and overuse injuries will occur if you utilize poor posture and overstride on the treadmill. Working on core stability, alignment, and posture will help avoid injuries and muscular aches.

Speak with a Personal Trainer

While apps and printed instructions might help you learn the perfect technique, nothing beats having an expert look at your form. Hire a personal trainer for a few sessions to ensure you do the routines correctly. It's an excellent investment; a personal trainer might be the most valuable safety item.

A trainer will monitor your technique to ensure you are not stressing your lower back or troublesome joints. A trainer will gradually increase your workout length and intensity, providing the optimum training result with the least chance of injury. During weight lifting, a trainer will also serve as a spotter.

Use Caution When Using Equipment

Tripping over something lying about is one of the most serious dangers of a gym accident. Clear the area of any things that you could trip over while moving. Also, keep in mind that the equipment is intended for knowledgeable adults.

Treadmills, exercise cycles, and weight machines all include moving elements that can pinch and crush your fingers and toes if you're not careful. Most gyms do not allow children in the training area, no matter how well-supervised they are.

Finally, ensure that pins and collars on weight machines and barbells are utilized appropriately. Be aware of who is working out around you and what motions they are doing so you may avoid getting in their way.

Train with a Friend

Working out alone at a gym is a good idea. It would be ideal if you could call on a friend or a staff member in case of an injury or a medical emergency. Working out with a partner might provide you with two sets of eyes on any emerging issues.

Encourage one another to drink, breathe properly, and rid the training area of obstructions. Be each other's safety and exercise partners.

If you lift weights, your partner should be able to detect you, which means they should be able to grasp the weight if your muscles fail throughout the activity. Many gyms require individuals lifting weights to have a spotter nearby. This is especially prevalent among barbell lifters, who may dump the weight on themselves if they attempt to lift one time too many.

Maintaining and improving your health is as simple as sticking to a fitness regimen and getting lots of physical activity. Gyms provide a wealth of equipment and assistance for various training activities. However, there are dangers to employing high-duty weights and equipment.

Following the safety rules and suggestions outlined above will enhance your safety and lower your risk of accidents and injuries. As usual, consult your healthcare practitioner before beginning any new workout regimen.

CHAPTER 4: BASIC WEIGHTLIFTING FOR BEGINNERS

The major weight training suggestion is to focus on many body motions, including several joints and muscles. This will allow you to use as many muscle fibers as possible. Joint exercises such as squats and push-ups are examples of such movement. These will significantly strengthen your legs, elbows, and core. Let's go through some weight-lifting training strategies that work:

To balance your workout, use push and pull movements. Balancing exercises can help you build your muscles evenly and lower your risk of injury.

To optimize and prevent damage, make sure you do each exercise correctly. Determine whether you want to develop your strength, muscle mass, or endurance, and create a full-proof training schedule accordingly.

Avoid working out the same muscle group twice in a row. Assist your body in recovering after each training session.

BENEFITS

Weight training has several advantages, and many people find it beneficial in different ways. Here are a few of our favorite reasons why you should incorporate weight training into your fitness routine:

Improved strength: With constant exercise, you should notice significant gains in the weight you can lift, push, or raise. Not only will you feel better at the gym, but you'll also see the benefit of your everyday exercises and confidence in your talents and power. To emphasize strength, perform fewer reps with heavier weights.

Weight training in the gym can help you in your daily life outside of the gym, such as being able to carry heavy items (great for grocery shopping and moving!), walking up stairs, or supporting improvements in other sports and activities like running, football, rowing, or tennis.

Build muscle: Consistently lifting weights over time can help expand the size of your muscles, enhancing strength and changing the look of your body - which is why bodybuilders choose this training strategy. Weight training allows you to target the muscles you want to grow by choosing the right exercises. Not everyone is trained to modify their looks or body composition. Still, weight training is essential if you want to bulk up or tone specific regions of your body.

Strengthen your bones: After age 30, you begin to lose bone density. Putting strain on your bones helps them to stay strong and reduces the likelihood of injury.

Better posture: Weight training that targets the entire body can help to strengthen regions like the back, shoulders, and core, allowing you to sit and stand more upright and improve your posture and stance.

Help with weight loss: When you lose weight, some of the weight you lose is muscle mass. Because muscle serves to maintain and develop your body, you'll generally want to keep as much of it as possible when losing weight, so including weight training in your fitness regimen is a smart option. Furthermore, muscle mass can influence your basal metabolic rate, which affects how many calories you burn naturally at rest.

Maintaining strong leg and core muscles helps avoid weak and shaky limbs. Weight training can help us stay stronger on our feet and less prone to fall as we age. It can also assist in correcting any physical imbalances, so if one arm is stronger than the other, you can undertake exercises to strengthen the weaker limb.

Reduce anxiety: Studies have indicated that weight training, in particular, can help reduce depressive symptoms. Aside from the confidence-boosting benefits of witnessing obvious changes in your talents and physique, weight training also helps generate mood-enhancing endorphins, which may alleviate anxiety and enhance your mental well-being.

WEIGHTLIFTING EXERCISES

Weightlifting is a popular and efficient type of resistance training in which weights are lifted to increase strength and power. For ages, yoga has been a cornerstone of fitness and sports training, and its benefits extend beyond the gym, significantly benefiting daily life and general health. In this post, we'll review some fundamental weightlifting exercises at the heart of every strength training program.

Squat

The squat is often regarded as the apex of all weightlifting exercises. It primarily targets lower-body muscles such as the quadriceps, hamstrings, glutes, and calves. It also works the core muscles and delivers a full-body exercise.

To squat, do the following:

- Place your feet shoulder-width apart.
- Maintain a straight back and a raised chest.
- Begin by bringing your hips back and bending your knees.
- Reduce your weight until your thighs parallel the ground, or go deeper if possible.
- To get back up, push through your heels.

Squats are important not just for increasing leg strength but also for improving balance and mobility. Front and overhead squat variations present extra difficulties and target different muscle areas.

Deadlift

Another important weightlifting exercise that focuses on the posterior chain, which comprises the lower back, glutes, and hamstrings, is the deadlift. It also strengthens the forearms, grip strength, and upper back.

To complete a deadlift, follow these steps:

- Place a barbell in front of you and stand with your feet hip-width apart.
- Lower your body by bending at the hips and knees and gripping the barbell slightly outside your knees.
- Maintain a flat back and a raised chest.
- Lift the barbell by pushing through your heels straightening your hips and knees.
- Stand up straight, shoulders back, and hips completely stretched.

Deadlifts are an excellent workout for increasing general strength and functional fitness. To avoid damage, starting with lesser weights and gradually raising the load as your technique improves is critical.

Bench Pressing

The bench press is the most well-known upper-body weightlifting exercise. It focuses on the chest, shoulders, and triceps while exercising the back and core for stability.

To complete a bench press, follow these steps:

- Lie on your back with your feet flat on a bench.
- Grip the barbell with your hands slightly wider than shoulder-width apart.
- Bend your elbows and lower the barbell to your chest.
- Return the barbell to its starting position until your arms are completely extended.

Bench presses are a cornerstone in most strength training regimens because they are effective for developing chest and upper body strength. Bench presses that are inclined or declined can target different chest regions.

Overhead Printing

The military press, commonly known as the overhead press, works the shoulders, triceps, and upper back. It's a functional workout that can aid with shoulder stability and strength.

To complete an overhead press, follow these steps:

- Place your feet shoulder-width apart.
- Hold a barbell or dumbbell at shoulder height with your palms facing front.
- Extend your arms overhead until they are completely stretched.
- Return the weight to shoulder height.

The overhead press is necessary for developing strong and stable shoulders, which are needed for various daily tasks and sports.

Pull-Up

Pull-ups, while not a classic weightlifting exercise, are a good bodyweight activity for increasing upper body strength, particularly in the back and biceps.

To do a pull-up, follow these steps:

- Hands facing away from your body, hang from a horizontal bar.
- Pull your body up till your chin is higher than the bar.
- Controlfully lower your body back down.

Pull-ups are difficult, but they provide considerable advantages for upper body strength and may be customized to your fitness level.

Rowing with Barbells

The barbell row is vital for targeting upper back muscles such as the lats, rhomboids, and biceps.

To do a barbell row, follow these steps:

- Hold a barbell with a shoulder-width grip and stand with your feet hip-width apart.
- Maintain a flat back by bending at the hips and knees.
- Squeeze your shoulder blades together as you pull the barbell towards your lower ribcage.
- Controllably lower the barbell back down.

Barbell rows enhance posture, strengthen the back, and contribute to a well-rounded upper body.

Jerk and Clean

The clean and jerk is a weightlifting exercise combining two separate motions: the clean and the jerk. This challenging exercise needs explosive strength, quickness, and skill while engaging many muscle groups.

- To do a clean and jerk:
- Begin with the barbell on the ground and clean it up to shoulder height.
- Then, pull the weight above while stretching your hips and legs and driving the barbell upward.
- Finish by standing tall with the barbell completely stretched overhead.

Clean and jerks are difficult but extremely effective exercises for improving total-body power, explosiveness, and coordination.

Snatch

The snatch is another Olympic weightlifting exercise in which a barbell is lifted continuously from the ground to overhead. It necessitates great speed, strength, skill, and several muscle groups.

Snatching is done as follows:

- Begin by placing the barbell on the ground and taking a broad grip.
- Lift the barbell explosively, stretching your hips and knees and bringing it overhead in a single stroke.

- Finish with the barbell overhead locked out and your body in a secure position.

Snatches are one of the most difficult weightlifting exercises, yet they significantly impact general athleticism, strength, and coordination.

Lunges using Dumbbells

Dumbbell lunges target the quadriceps, hamstrings, glutes, and calves while increasing balance and stability.

To do dumbbell lunges, follow these steps:

- Hold a dumbbell on either side of your body.
- Step forward and lower your body until both knees are bent at 90-degree angles.
- To return to the beginning position, push via the front heel.
- For each repeat, alternate legs.

Dumbbell lunges provide a unilateral movement pattern that addresses muscular imbalances and improves functional fitness.

Deadlift in Romania

The Romanian deadlift is a version of the standard deadlift that emphasizes the hamstrings and lower back. It's a terrific workout for increasing posterior chain strength and flexibility.

To do a Romanian deadlift, follow these steps:

- Hold a barbell or dumbbell in front of your thighs while standing with your feet hip-width apart.
- Maintaining a flat back and slightly bent knees, flex at the hips and reduce your weight to the ground.
- Lower the weight until you feel a stretch in your hamstrings, then extend your hips to return to the starting position.

Romanian deadlifts are good for hamstring strength, which can help prevent injuries and enhance athletic performance.

Push-Up

The push-up is a traditional bodyweight exercise that works the chest, shoulders, triceps, and core muscles. It's a flexible workout that can be tailored to various fitness levels.

To do a push-up, follow these steps:

- Begin in a plank stance, and hands shoulder-width apart.
- Bend your elbows and lower your body until your chest is barely above the ground.
- Return your body to the beginning position.

Push-ups are an important exercise for developing upper-body strength and are frequently employed as a fitness test.

The Russian Twist

The Russian twist is a core-building exercise that works the obliques and abdominal muscles. It is done sitting on the ground, either with or without weight.

To add a Russian twist:

Sit on the ground with your knees bent and your feet flat.

- Lean back gently while maintaining a straight back.
- Hold a weight or medicine ball in front of your chest with both hands.
- Twist your body to the left and right, tapping the weight close to your hip on the ground.

Russian twists improve core stability and rotational strength, which is vital for various sports and activities.

Swing a kettlebell

The kettlebell swing is a dynamic exercise that works the posterior chain (glutes, hamstrings, and lower back). It also works the core and the shoulders.

To do a kettlebell swing, follow these steps:

- Stand with your feet shoulder-width apart and a kettlebell in front of you with both hands.
- Maintain a flat back by bending at the hips and knees.
- Swing the kettlebell back and forth between your legs.
- Extend your hips explosively and swing the kettlebell to shoulder height while maintaining your arms straight.

Kettlebell swings are excellent for increasing explosive hip power and cardiovascular fitness.

Plank

The plank is a basic yet powerful core-strengthening exercise that works the abs, lower back, and shoulders.

A plank is performed as follows.

- Begin by doing a push-up with your elbows just beneath your shoulders.
- Maintain a straight line from head to heels by activating your core muscles.
- Maintain appropriate form and hold the posture for as long as you can.

Planks are a basic exercise for developing core stability, which is necessary for general strength and posture.

Box Jumping

Box leaps are a plyometric exercise that emphasizes explosive lower body power. They work on quadriceps, hamstrings, glutes, coordination, and balance.

To do a box jump, follow these steps:

- Place yourself in front of a strong box or platform.
- Bend your hips and knees, then jump onto the box explosively, landing lightly with bent knees.
- Step or leap back to the starting position after standing straight on the box.

Box jumps are a great supplement to any strength and conditioning program, particularly for athletes aiming to improve their explosive power.

CHAPTER 5: BEGINNER-FRIENDLY WORKOUT ROUTINES

Developing an exercise regimen for beginners is an important step in laying a solid foundation for fitness. To avoid injuries, whether new to exercising or returning to a regimen after a hiatus, it's critical to start carefully and focus on appropriate techniques. This book will give beginners sample full-body and split exercise routines, emphasizing the need for warm-ups and cool-downs to guarantee a safe and productive training experience.

Warm-Ups and Cool-Downs Are Important

Before we get into training programs, it's important to grasp the importance of warm-ups and cool-downs:

Warm-up: A thorough warm-up is critical for preparing your body for the workout. It gradually raises your heart rate, circulation, and body temperature, which aids in the relaxation of muscles and joints. A solid warm-up also mentally prepares you for the next activity, lowering your chance of injury. Warm-up activities should take 5-10 minutes, including brisk walking, running, jumping jacks, or dynamic stretches.

Cool-Down:

It is just as vital to cool down after a workout as to warm up. It allows your heart rate and respiration to recover normally while preventing muscular tightness and stiffness. A typical cool-down comprises static stretching activities that target the muscles engaged throughout the activity. Focus on deep, regulated breathing while holding each stretch for 15-30 seconds. Now that we've covered warm-ups and cool-downs let's look at some basic exercise routines:

Full-Body Workout Routine Example

A full-body exercise works out many muscle groups in a single session, making it a good choice for beginners. Repeat this program 2-3 times weekly, with at least one day between.

(5–10 minutes) Warm-up

Walking at a moderate speed increases heart rate and circulation.

Arm Circles: Stand with your arms outstretched to the sides and circularly move your arms. Begin with tiny circles and progressively expand their size.

Leg Swings: Grab a firm surface and slowly swing one leg forth and backward. Rep with the other leg.

Workout for the Whole Body (Do 2-3 sets of 10-15 repetitions for each exercise.)

Squats using your body weight: Stand with your feet shoulder-width apart and squat down as if sitting in a chair. Maintain a straight back and a raised chest.

Push-Ups (Knee Push-Ups for Beginners): Place your hands shoulder-width apart on the floor, then bend your elbows to drop your chest to the ground. Maintain a straight line with your body.

Rows using dumbbells (or resistance bands): Use resistance bands or a dumbbell in each hand. Pull the weights towards your hips while bending and keeping your back straight.

Plank: Similar to a push-up, but with your weight on your forearms rather than your hands. Maintain a straight line from head to heels.

Lie on your back with your knees bent and your feet flat on the floor for Glute Bridges. Squeeze your glutes as you lift your hips off the ground.

Dumbbell Lunges (or Bodyweight Lunges): Use a dumbbell or your body weight in each hand. Step forward with one leg, bend both knees, and lower yourself until your front thigh is parallel to the ground.

Lie on your back with your hands behind your head for Bicycle Crunches. While extending your left leg, bring your left elbow and right knee together. In a pedaling action, alternate sides.

Cooling time (5-10 minutes)

Standing Quadriceps Stretch: Stand on one leg and slowly pull your opposing ankle toward your glutes.

Stand facing a wall, plant one foot behind you, toes pointing forward, and press your heel into the ground.

Stretch your hamstrings by sitting on the ground with one leg extended and the other bowed. Extend your hand toward your outstretched foot.

Stretch your triceps by extending one arm above, bending your elbow, and reaching your hand down your back. Gently press your bent elbow with your opposing hand.

Sit on your heels, legs apart, and extend your arms forward, lowering your chest to the ground.

Split Workout Routine Example

A split exercise plan focuses on distinct muscle groups on separate days, allowing for more concentrated training. This workout is appropriate for beginners who want to focus on different muscle groups on different days. Perform this practice three to four times weekly, with at least one day between workouts.

Warm-up (5-10 minutes) - Perform the same exercises as in the full-body regimen.

First Day: Upper Body

Triceps and chest:

Push-ups (or Knee Push-Ups for Beginners): 2-3 sets of 10-15 repetitions.

Bench Press with Dumbbells (or Push-Ups): 2-3 sets of 10-15 repetitions.

Tricep Dips: 2-3 sets of 10-15 repetitions (on a solid surface).

Second Day: Lower Body

Glutes and legs:

Squats with bodyweight: 2-3 sets of 10-15 repetitions.

Dumbbell Lunges (or Bodyweight Lunges): 2-3 sets of 10-15 repetitions.

2-3 sets of 10-15 repetitions on the glute bridges.

DAY 3: REST OR LIGHT ACTIVITY (FOR EXAMPLE, WALKING OR YOGA)

4th Day: Upper Body

Biceps and back:

Rows with dumbbells (or resistance bands): 2-3 sets of 10-15 repetitions.

Bicep Curls: 2-3 sets of 10-15 repetitions (using dumbbells or resistance bands).

Hold the plank position for 30-60 seconds.

5th Day: Lower Body

Core and Legs:

Leg Raises: Lie on your back, straighten your legs, and lift them toward the sky. Lower them back down without allowing them to make contact with the earth. 2-3 sets of 10-15 repetitions.

Russian Twists (dumbbells or water bottles): Sit on the ground with your knees bent, and while holding the weight, rotate your body to either side. 2-3 sets of 15-20 repetitions on each side.

Lean against a wall with your knees bent at a 90-degree angle and hold for as long as possible.

Cool-down (5-10 minutes) - Repeat the full-body program.

Success Hints

Consistency is essential: Maintain your exercise program and progressively raise the intensity as you gain strength and familiarity with the workouts.

Maintain proper form during each exercise to minimize the chance of injury and optimize benefits.

Progressive overload: As you develop, increase the weights or resistance to test your muscles and progress.

Pay attention to your body: Consult a healthcare practitioner or a fitness trainer if your discomfort goes beyond normal muscular soreness.

Stay hydrated by drinking lots of water before, during, and after workouts.

Rest and recovery: Sleep enough and give your body time to recuperate between exercises.

Nutrition: A well-balanced diet rich in nutrient-dense meals is vital for achieving your fitness objectives.

CHAPTER 6: CARDIOVASCULAR EXERCISES

Regular aerobic activity, as part of a heart-healthy lifestyle, can not only lower your resting blood pressure and heart rate, but these simple adjustments can also mean your heart doesn't have to work as hard all the time. Regular exercise also helps increase cholesterol levels while decreasing blood fats.

Cardio improves more than just your heart. Indeed, studies show that obtaining adequate cardiovascular activity may help you live longer.

How Cardio May Help your Brain

Cardiovascular activity can help preserve your brain as you age. According to one study, physical activity may lessen the incidence of dementia regardless of age. Other advantages may include:

- Increasing blood flow and lowering the risk of stroke.
- Improving memory and cognition.
- Combating the aging-related loss in brain function.
- Defending your brain from Alzheimer's disease.

How Cardio May Help Your Joints

We've all felt a little shaky at times. While relaxing may be tempting, the greatest way to enhance joint health is to begin active. Cardiovascular exercise is beneficial:

Combat osteoporosis and lower your risk of hip fracture.

Manage arthritic pain while maintaining range of motion.

How Aerobics May Help your Skin

Being active, regardless of how you move, helps enhance circulation, leading to smoother, healthier skin. In practice, this translates to:

Improved blood flow to your cells, particularly those on your face. This helps to minimize age symptoms and enhance your complexion.

Reduced stress helps to keep chronic skin disorders like eczema at bay.

How Cardio May Help Your Muscles

"Wait a minute," you might be thinking, "strength training and cardio are two completely different things!"

You are correct. However, maintaining your muscles healthy is more than just making them stronger.

Working your heart and other body muscles during cardiac exercise boosts oxygen flow to the entire body, allowing all muscles to perform harder and more efficiently. Ordinary cardiac exercise permits your muscles to adapt to an increased burden over time, making ordinary tasks appear simpler.

How Cardio Can Help Your Digestion

Peristalsis is accelerated. Cardio, as previously said, allows your muscles to operate harder. This includes the muscles that propel peristalsis, or food movement, through your digestive system. Don't perform high-intensity exercise after eating, or you may have cramps or lightheadedness.

Improves blood sugar control. Your pancreas is an organ that aids digestion by converting the food you ingest into energy. Staying active improves blood sugar management, minimizes stress on this important organ, and lowers your risk of developing Type 2 diabetes.

Aids in the regulation of your gut bacteria. According to studies, exercise may help you have a broad and abundant population of beneficial bacteria in your gut.

How Aerobics Can Help Your Lungs

"Physical activity benefits your lungs as well," "Cardio helps decrease how frequently you have to breathe as exercise improves and can lead to reductions in fatigue and shortness of breath in chronic lung problems like asthma."

Weight reduction

Regular cardiac activity leads to safe weight loss and a healthy diet. A healthy weight not only reduces your risk of developing diseases such as diabetes, some cancers, and heart disease, but it also allows your body to circulate blood more freely. Less sitting time and increased physical exercise also aid in weight maintenance by burning more calories throughout the day.

Boosts energy

There's a reason you feel so good after a workout. Cardio activity boosts your energy by generating endorphins, which provide you with greater, longer-lasting energy throughout the day.

Enhances sleep

When it comes to hitting the covers, the last thing you want to do after a long, hectic day is struggle to fall asleep. The good news is that aerobics increases REM sleep and helps you fall asleep faster.

However, there is a catch. "Make sure to avoid rigorous exercise too close to bed, or you could be left too energized to count sheep due to having too much adrenaline circulating,"

Improves your immune system

Less stress + more sleep + improved blood and oxygen flow to cells = a stronger, more effective immune system. When you get sick, there is evidence that low-intensity exercise can help you recover quicker from some diseases by reducing your symptoms.

One major caveat, however: always include downtime in your training plan. Too much high-intensity exercise regularly might impair your immune system.

Reduces your chances of falling

It's a frustrating truth that our danger of falling – and catastrophic harm – increases as we age and our mobility declines.

We usually think of strength and balance workouts rather than cardio when considering fall prevention. However, you profit from all three. After all, your balance and strength are only as good as your endurance.

CARDIO EXERCISES

1. Walking with Power

Starting a power walking program can help you stay active, boost your lifespan, and help you lose weight. You may cover several miles in this low-impact type of aerobics by ramping up the pace and walking with purpose. In just two weeks of power walking practice, you may see major advantages ranging from lower blood pressure to stronger leg muscles. Beginners should start with 10 minutes per day and gradually increase the time they walk by 5 minutes each day until they can walk for 30 minutes.

Some power walking tips:

- Keep your head upright and your chin in a neutral position to maintain excellent posture. With each step, engage your core and glutes.
- Longer strides should be avoided in favor of shorter, smoother steps.
- Begin by striking the ground with your heel, then rolling onto the ball of your foot, and lastly, pushing off your toes.
- Engage your arms for a total-body workout and an additional 10% calorie burn. Bend your elbows and swing your arms in step with your feet.

Jogging

Running is a great entrance point into fitness for novices since it is free and does not require any special equipment. Running and jogging are both good kinds of aerobic exercise. Studies have shown running to lower the risk of obesity, high blood pressure, heart disease, cancer, type 2 diabetes, and other diseases. If you're a newbie, starting slowly with brisk walking, jogging, and running is best. Allow at least six weeks to build up to regular jogging, and remember to warm up fully before you go and do some easy stretches to cool down after your run.

Some running tips:

- Keep your strides short and rapid. Maintain a neutral head posture and forward gaze. Run on the balls of your feet instead of your heels or toes.
- Our fitness experts recommend gently moving your shoulders forward and backward every mile to relieve stiffness while running longer distances.
- Invest in high-quality running equipment, such as solid running shoes. If you're jogging outside, workout gear and accessories with reflective elements on the front and back are vital for increasing your visibility to vehicles and other pedestrians.
- Because running is a repeated activity in the same plane of motion, it is critical to include rest days to avoid overtraining and to supplement your running program with other activities, such as strength training.

ROWING

Rowing is a terrific, low-impact type of exercise that gives an effective method to break a sweat. Indoor rowing machines are gaining popularity since they work practically every muscle in the body. This type of exercise is more efficient than cycling or jogging since you push with your legs and pull with your arms. It's also an excellent starting point for people with joint problems.

Some rowing tips:

- Keep your knees straight with each stroke, and avoid bending them to the side.
- Keep your shoulders from hunching. Sit up straight, shoulders relaxed, and shoulders away from your ears.
- Maintain a firm grasp on the handle so it doesn't slip out of your hands, but don't over-grip since this might cause forearm fatigue.
- The rowing technique requires core engagement, so activate this important muscle group with each stroke.

CYCLING

Indoor and outdoor cycling are fantastic low-impact cardio forms suitable for people of all fitness levels. You may vary the intensity with both speed and resistance, providing for training diversity and efficiency. Exercise bikes are an excellent addition to any home gym, ranging from high-end smart bikes with guided courses to simple recumbent cycles for a great workout. Indoor cycling has been demonstrated to increase aerobic capacity and blood pressure.

Some cycling tips:

- Positioning is essential for a smooth and effective ride. Handlebars on indoor cycling cycles should be high enough so that you don't feel any pressure on your back.
- Seating should be positioned so the legs are slightly bent during the pedal stroke. Position the seat so the front pedal is below your knee if it adjusts horizontally.
- If you have discomfort in the front of your knee, raise your seat; if you have pain in the rear of your knee, lower your seat.
- Your elbows should be slightly bent, your back should be straight, and your core should be engaged.
- According to our experts, investing in a decent pair of cycling shoes helps you to become one with your bike and have a more smooth and controlled pedal stroke.

SWIMMING

Moving your entire body against water resistance provides excellent aerobic exercise that is also enjoyable. Swimming may help you increase endurance, tone your muscles, and keep your heart rate up while reducing joint impact. According to studies, it's also a calm and serene exercise that can help relieve stress and enhance mood. Many types of cardio may be challenging for those with arthritis, but swimming can assist in improving the usage of damaged joints without exacerbating symptoms.

Some swimming tips:

- Ensure you have a nice set of goggles and a quality sports swimsuit.
- As you swim, maintain a neutral head posture by keeping your head aligned with the rest of your body and staring down toward the pool's bottom.
- During your swim workout, aim for tiny, consistent kicks. Ensure your hand and arm do not cross your body's midline as you go through the water.
- Make each breath count, and exhale completely before taking a rapid, deep breath on the side.

GUIDANCE ON SETTING CARDIO WORKOUT GOALS

Setting specific and attainable cardio workout objectives is critical for remaining motivated and keeping track of your progress. Here are some pointers to help you set effective cardio training goals:

Determine Your Motivation:

Recognize why you want to include cardio activities in your schedule. Is it for weight loss, cardiovascular health, stamina, stress reduction, or something else? Knowing your motivation will assist you in setting appropriate objectives.

Begin with short-term objectives:

Begin with short-term goals you can complete in a few weeks or months. Achieving these goals will increase your self-esteem and motivation.

For example, if you're new to jogging, your first aim may be to jog for 10 minutes without stopping.

Increase the intensity and duration gradually:

Increase the intensity and duration of your aerobic exercises progressively as you reach your short-term goals. This gradual approach reduces the likelihood of burnout and overuse damage.

For example, if you aim to walk for 30 minutes every day and reach that goal, you can graduate to jogging for 30 minutes and, eventually, running for 30 minutes.

Set long-term objectives:

Long-term objectives give your fitness journey direction and purpose. They are frequently more difficult and require longer to complete.

A long-term objective may be to run a half marathon, bike 50 miles, or achieve a certain body fat percentage.

Monitor Your Progress:

Keep a workout log or track your progress with fitness apps and wearables. Details such as workout time, distance traveled, heart rate, and perceived exertion level should be recorded.

Examine your records on a regular basis to assess how far you've gone and where you might need to make changes.

Maintain your adaptability:

Be willing to adapt your goals if circumstances change. Life may be unexpected. Therefore, tailoring your objectives to your present position and talents is critical.

Treat Yourself:

Celebrate your accomplishments, no matter how minor they may appear. Rewards may reinforce positive actions, which can drive you to keep working toward your goals.

Seek assistance and accountability:

Share your objectives with a friend, family member, or gym companion who can offer encouragement and hold you responsible.

Joining a fitness group or class might help you stay motivated and connect with people with similar aims.

Seek Professional Advice:

Consider working with a professional personal trainer or a fitness coach if you're concerned about setting appropriate objectives or need advice on a specific fitness plan. They may offer specialized guidance and assist you in developing a customized training

BLAKE KEACH

routine.

CHAPTER 7: NUTRITION FOR GYM BEGINNERS

IMPORTANCE OF A BALANCED DIET TO SUPPORT FITNESS GOALS

Because it supplies the essential nutrients, energy, and fuel that your body needs to perform at its very best during exercises, recover efficiently afterward, and progress toward long-term fitness goals, a nutritionally sound diet is critical for facilitating the achievement of fitness objectives. The following is a list of numerous reasons why it is necessary to support your fitness objectives with a balanced diet:

Vitality for Physical Activity:

The major source of fuel for the body is comprised of carbohydrates. Your workouts must be fueled with carbs, and your energy levels must be maintained during exercise sessions. A balanced diet includes a sufficient quantity of carbohydrates. If you don't get enough carbs, you'll probably feel tired and unable to function as well as you might.

Maintenance and Development of Muscle:

Protein is essential for muscle growth, development, and maintenance: strength training and other resistance exercise cause microscopic tears to appear in the working muscle fibers. A diet high in protein supplies the amino acids required for the healing and development of these muscles, which in turn makes them stronger and more resilient.

Recuperation and Rebuilding:

Following exercise, your body needs specific nutrients to heal damaged tissue and restore glycogen levels. This recuperation process is helped by eating a balanced diet that includes vitamins, minerals, and antioxidants. This diet also helps reduce the chance of injuries and promotes general health and wellness.

Management of One's Weight:

Intake of calories may be controlled, which in turn assists in maintaining a healthy weight. Consuming a diet with suitable portions and a nutritional balance is vital if your fitness objectives include losing or maintaining your current weight. It can assist you in producing a calorie deficit, which is necessary for weight reduction and maintaining a healthy weight.

Performance at Its Highest Level:

Foods high in nutrients, such as fruits and vegetables, are good sources of the vitamins and minerals necessary for good health and well-being. Your performance may be improved by ensuring that your body performs well and that you have the stamina to sustain longer more intensive workouts. This can be accomplished by consuming the appropriate foods.

Water Intake:

A healthy diet must always focus on maintaining an appropriate level of fluids. During exercise, it is very important to drink plenty of water so that your temperature can be controlled, nutrients can be transported, and electrolyte balance can be preserved. Decreased performance, muscular cramps, and additional issues might result from dehydration.

Avoiding Fatigue and Cramps in Your Muscles:

Consuming adequate minerals, such as potassium, magnesium, and salt, is essential to avoid experiencing muscular cramps and weariness while engaging in physical activity. You can ensure that you obtain enough of these critical minerals by following a healthy diet that includes various foods.

Support for the Immune System:

Taking part in regular exercise lowers one's immunological defenses. A healthy, well-balanced diet high in antioxidants and vitamins, such as vitamins C and E, can help strengthen your immune system and lower the likelihood of becoming unwell or infected. This will enable you to maintain your normal exercise routine.

Sustainability Over the Long Term:

A diet that is both sustainable and effective in promoting healthy eating habits for the long term is called a balanced diet. It ensures you get a wide range of nutrients and prevents you from relying on restrictive diets, which can result in nutrient deficits and fatigue.

Psychological Fitness and the Drive to Win:

Consuming foods that are high in nutrients can have a beneficial effect on one's mood as well as their mental clarity. If you are psychologically healthy, you will have an easier time maintaining your motivation and staying devoted to the fitness objectives you have set for yourself.

BASIC NUTRITION TIPS FOR ENERGY AND RECOVERY

Providing energy for workouts and promoting recovery after that are significantly aided by proper nutrition. The following are some fundamental dietary pointers that can help you optimize your energy and increase your recovery:

For Energy Before Physical Activity:

Carbohydrates: Carbohydrates are the major energy source used by your body. In order to give your body continuous energy during your workout, consume complex carbohydrates such as whole grains (for example, oats, brown rice, and quinoa), fruits, and vegetables a few hours before you begin.

Hydration: Keeping yourself well hydrated is necessary to maintain your energy levels. Consume water at regular intervals throughout the day, and take into consideration eating a modest amount of water or a sports drink around thirty minutes before beginning physical activity, particularly for longer or more strenuous exercises.

Meals That Are Light and Well-Balanced: You should avoid eating large or heavy meals just before work because they might cause pain and gastrointestinal problems. Instead, go for a lunch or snack that is light and well-balanced, consisting of carbs, protein, and a tiny bit of healthy fat in the right proportions.

Snacks to Consume Before Working Out Some snacks to consume

before working out are a banana spread with almond butter, Greek yogurt mixed with berries, or whole-grain toast with avocado. These offer a balanced combination of carbs and protein to keep your energy levels up.

For Recovery After Physical Activity:

Consuming protein after exercise is essential for promoting muscle repair and development and should be a priority. Make it a goal to incorporate a source of lean protein into your meal or snack after your workout. Various options are available, including chicken, fish, eggs, tofu, and plant-based proteins like lentils and beans.

Carbs: Consuming carbs after exercise is the best way to replenish depleted glycogen levels. This aids in the regeneration of energy as well as the healing of muscles. Whole grains, sweet potatoes, or even a piece of fruit are great examples of ideal sources.

Hydration: After your workout, it is important to rehydrate your body by consuming water or a sports drink, particularly if you sweated substantially. Drink between 16 and 24 ounces of liquids for every pound of body weight lost due to activity. This serves as a basic guideline.

Antioxidants: Consuming foods that are high in antioxidants, such as berries, leafy greens, and citrus fruits, can assist in the fight against oxidative stress and inflammation that are brought on by physical activity.

Include healthy fats in your post-exercise meal, such as avocados, almonds, and olive oil, to improve nutrient absorption and general recovery. This will help you get the most out of your workout.

When it comes to timing, the optimal time to consume a well-balanced meal or snack after an exercise is between 30 minutes and two hours. During this time frame, your body is most sensitive to absorbing nutrients.

Additional Suggestions for Maintaining Your Energy and Recovering:

Pay Attention to Your Body: Pay attention to the signs your body is giving you that it is hungry, and adapt your diet appropriately. If you engage in a particularly taxing workout, you could require a greater quantity of calories and nutrients to facilitate your body's recovery.

Maintain a constant eating schedule and fuelling approach to ensure your body gets the nutrients it needs for energy and recovery. This will guarantee that your body is able to stay consistent.

Sugar may cause energy levels to rise and collapse, so limit your consumption of sugary foods and beverages as much as possible. Carbohydrates are necessary for energy production, but consuming too much sugar can cause energy levels to swing wildly.

Before choosing supplements, discussing your options with a qualified medical practitioner or licensed dietician is important. Certain nutritional supplements, such as protein powder or branched-chain amino acids, may, in certain instances, be useful in pursuing particular fitness goals.

You should strive to maintain a well-balanced diet of various nutrient-rich foods. Not only does this help your energy levels and recovery, but it also makes a contribution to your general health and well-being.

MISCONCEPTIONS ABOUT DIETING AND EXERCISE

Misconceptions about nutrition and exercise can result in frustration, false expectations, and difficulty adopting and maintaining a healthy lifestyle. Let me address some of these myths:

1: Crash Diets Work for Long-Term Weight Loss

Crash diets, which entail severe calorie restriction or the exclusion of whole food categories, might first result in quick weight reduction. They are, however, often unsustainable and can be hazardous to your health. When most people resume their usual eating habits, they recover their lost weight. Making incremental, healthy modifications to your food and lifestyle is the key to long-term weight loss.

2: It Is Possible to "Spot Reduce" Fat

Many individuals assume that performing certain workouts for specific body regions (for example, crunches for a flat stomach) can remove fat in those areas. Fat loss happens throughout the body when a calorie deficit is created through food and activity. It is impossible to lose weight in just one location.

3: To Lose Weight, you should eat as little as possible.

Reality: Extreme calorie restriction can slow your metabolism, induce muscle loss, and lead to vitamin shortages. It may also result in binge eating or other harmful eating habits. Consuming a suitable quantity of calories appropriate for your activity level, age, and gender while focusing on nutrient-dense meals is essential for weight reduction.

4: Exercise Alone Is Enough for Weight Loss

While exercise is important for general health and can help with weight loss, it is not a stand-alone solution for considerable weight loss. Diet plays a larger part in weight management. A calorie deficit must be created by combining food and activity to lose weight.

5: All Calories Are Created Equal

When it comes to nutrition, not all calories are created equal. It is important to consider the quality of the calories you consume. Nutrient-dense meals such as fruits, vegetables, lean meats, and whole grains supply necessary vitamins and minerals. However, despite being abundant in calories, sugary and highly processed foods might lead to health concerns.

6: To Succeed, Weight Loss should be Accomplished Quickly

Reality: Rapid weight reduction sometimes necessitates drastic procedures that are difficult to maintain. A better and more practical strategy is to aim for a weekly weight loss of 1-2 pounds. Slow and steady progress is more likely to provide long-term effects.

7: Exercise Is Only for Losing Weight

Reality: Exercise has several health advantages in addition to weight reduction. It improves cardiovascular health, muscle strength, mood, and energy levels and lowers the risk of chronic illnesses. Concentrating simply on exercise for weight loss ignores these other substantial advantages.

8: To Be Healthy, You Must Adhere to a Specific Diet Trend

There is no such thing as a one-size-fits-all diet that works for everyone. Healthy eating habits differ from individual to person. Selecting a diet that fits your interests and lifestyle while satisfying your nutritional demands is critical. A well-balanced diet rich in whole foods is a wonderful place to start.

9: Supplements Can Substitute for a Healthy Diet

While certain supplements can be useful, they should not be taken in place of a well-balanced diet. Whole foods include a wide variety of nutrients that interact together synergistically in ways that pills cannot.

10: Fitness Is Only About Appearance

Reality: Fitness is more than simply looking good. Overall health, strength, flexibility, and endurance are all included. Concentrating entirely on looks can lead to unrealistic body standards and neglect other important components of well-being.

CHAPTER 8: STAYING CONSISTENT AND OVERCOMING CHALLENGES

It can be not easy to keep motivated and consistent while you are on a journey to improve your health and fitness, but there are several tactics that you can use to help you stay on track and accomplish your objectives:

1. Establish Objectives That Are Both Specific and Clear:

Define your fitness goals very specifically. Please ensure they are SMART, which is specific, measurable, attainable, relevant, and time-bound. Having a distinct sense of purpose can assist you in maintaining your motivation.

2. Formulate a Strategy:

Create a planned strategy for both your workouts and your diet. Having a strategy in place helps alleviate decision fatigue and ensures that you are aware of what must be completed on a daily basis.

3. Investigate your "Why":

Determine the more fundamental motivations that drive you to achieve your fitness objectives. When things get difficult, having a clear idea of why you want to achieve your goals may be a powerful source of drive.

4. Get Going Gently and Step by Step:

Refrain from attempting to take on too much too quickly. You should begin with doable workouts, and as your strength and stamina improve, you should progressively increase the intensity, duration, or frequency of your workouts.

5. Ensure That It Is Enjoyable:

Pick out pursuits that you are excited about. It doesn't matter if the activity is dancing, hiking, swimming, or playing on a team—if you're having fun with it, you're more likely to continue doing it.

6. Look for a Person to Hold You Accountable:

Exercise with a friend or sign up for a class or group activity at a gym. Accountability partners can encourage and help one another while also providing support.

7. Keep Tabs on Your Advancement:

Maintaining a fitness diary is a great way to keep track of your exercises, diet, and how you're feeling overall. Honor all of your accomplishments, no matter how minor they may seem.

8. Make Use of Modern Technology

Using fitness wearables and apps may assist you in keeping track of your progress, establish reminders, and remain focused on your objectives.

9. Create a Regular Schedule:

Develop a routine for your physical activity that fits in with the rest of your day. The more ingrained it is in your habit, the less likely you will skip it.

10. Ensure That Your Expectations Are Realistic:

It is important to remember that growth may only sometimes occur linearly and that there will be obstacles to overcome. Have patience with yourself and keep your attention on the bigger picture.

11. Give Yourself a Treat:

Reward yourself for your accomplishments with things that are not food. For instance, get yourself new exercise gear, treat yourself to a day at the spa, or treat yourself to a movie night.

12. Keep Yourself Informed:

Make it a habit to regularly educate yourself on health, exercise, and nutrition topics. More information might give you the power to make better decisions and keep you motivated.

13. Picture yourself succeeding:

Imagine that you have already accomplished all of your objectives. The power of visualization may be a potent motivator that assists you in maintaining your concentration on your goals.

14. Avoiding and Overcoming Plateaus:

In any fitness quest, reaching a plateau is perfectly acceptable. When you reach this point, consider switching up your workout program, trying out some new activities, or getting advice from a fitness expert.

15. Make a habit of showing compassion to yourself:

Be gentle to yourself at all times, especially on the difficult days. Avoid being too critical of yourself since doing so might make you feel unmotivated. Keep in mind that these kinds of things happen to everyone.

16. Maintain Your Adaptability:

There is no telling what will happen in life. Refrain from beating yourself up if you occasionally skip a workout or select foods less beneficial to your health. Find your footing again and let go of any guilt.

17. Seek Out Assistance:

If you need assistance or guidance, do not hesitate to ask for it or seek it from fitness professionals, certified dietitians, or therapists. They are able to offer insightful advice and dependable help.

18. Remain Consistent with a Few Steps at a Time:

On days when your motivation is low, make a pact with yourself to complete only a small portion of your workout or to make just one healthy option. Taking that initial step can frequently pave the way to a more comprehensive workout or improved dietary decisions.

COMMON CHALLENGES FACED BY BEGINNERS

When starting a new health and wellness practice or embarking on a quest to improve one's fitness level, novices frequently confront several typical obstacles. The following is a list of some of these difficulties, as well as some advice on how to overcome them:

1. A failure to motivate oneself:

The Obstacle:

It can be not easy to find the desire to begin a new fitness regimen and maintain it over time, especially when the consequences of the exercise are not seen right away.

The answer is:

Determine your "why" and ensure your goals are clear and significant. Bring back to memory all of the reasons you desire to get in better shape. Imagine yourself succeeding, and give yourself positive reinforcement whenever you reach a new goal.

2. Stress and an Excessive Amount of Information:

The Obstacle:

Beginners may need help navigating the abundance of information, meal plans, and exercise routines available in the health and fitness business.

The answer is:

Begin with the fundamentals. Pick a straightforward regimen for your workouts, and put most of your attention on eating healthfully. As you gain confidence and experience, gradually introduce more components into the mix. If you need direction, go to a nutritionist or a fitness expert.

3. Expectations that are not Realistic:

The Obstacle:

Some newcomers to a field have unrealistic expectations about how quickly they will see results and become disheartened when their development is slower than expected.

The answer is:

Establish attainable and reasonable objectives, and recognize that sustainable improvement takes time. We should not just focus on the end goal but also on the tiny triumphs we achieve along the road and celebrate them.

4. A Failure to Acquire Knowledge:

The Obstacle:

People starting in the fitness world might need help understanding appropriate exercise forms, nutrition, or how to design an efficient training routine.

The answer is:

Get some formal training. You may educate yourself about fitness and nutrition by reading authoritative books, enrolling in online classes, or working with a personal trainer or fitness coach who can guide and teach you the essentials.

5. Restrictions Placed on Time:

The Obstacle:

Finding the time to maintain healthy habits like exercising regularly and preparing nutritious meals can be challenging for people with busy schedules.

The answer is:

Make taking care of your body a priority by including time in your schedule for working, exercising, and preparing meals. Even relatively brief workouts that are intensely effective and straightforward, nutritious meals might make a difference. If your nights are often hectic, think about working out early in the morning or over lunch.

6. Inadequate Support from Social Groups:

The Obstacle:

It might be disappointing when friends and family don't support or encourage you in what you're doing.

The answer is:

Share your aspirations with those you care about and solicit their assistance. If you want to meet others who share your interests and goals, you should look into finding a workout partner or joining fitness programs or organizations.

7. The dread of being judged:

The Obstacle:

When they exercise in public or at a gym, some newcomers worry that they will be evaluated or experience feelings of self-consciousness.

The answer is:

Keep in mind that everyone has to begin somewhere and that the majority of individuals at the gym are preoccupied with their exercises. Choose to exercise in settings that make you feel at ease, such as working out at home or when the gym is less busy.

8. Continuities and Regressions:

The Obstacle:

In pursuing physical fitness, it is usual to experience plateaus and failures, which can be discouraging.

The answer is:

Recognize and accept that reaching a plateau is a natural and necessary progress element. You may overcome plateaus by adjusting your nutrition or workouts as necessary, and you shouldn't let temporary failures deter you. Take advantage of these situations as learning and development opportunities.

9. The Danger of Injuries:

The Obstacle:

Those just starting may have to spend more time learning the correct exercise method, which raises the possibility of being hurt.

The answer is:

Make safety your priority by getting proper instruction and beginning with low-impact workouts. To lessen the likelihood of being hurt, you should begin by warming up and stretching. Consult a trained fitness expert for advice if you need help with what to do.

10. Inconsistency in Presentation:

The Obstacle Is:

Especially when life gets hectic, maintaining a consistent routine with one's workouts and a healthy diet may be challenging.

The Answer Is:

Make a plan you can keep, and then try to stick to it as much as possible. Consider employing accountability tactics such as working out with a friend, setting reminders for yourself, or keeping a fitness journal to track your progress.

The key to keeping your motivation up and reaching your health and fitness objectives is to keep track of your progress and to have reasonable expectations for yourself. The following advice will assist you in keeping an accurate track of your progress and in setting goals that are within your reach:

ADVICE FOR MONITORING YOUR ADVANCEMENT

Maintain a Health and Fitness Journal:

Keep a log of your workouts, noting the exercises you perform, the number of sets and repetitions you complete, and the weights you use. Take careful mental notes on how you felt during and after each session.

Take the Suitable Measures:

Take frequent measurements of your body in certain areas (such as your waist, hips, chest, and arms) to monitor any changes in size or circumference.

Make Use of Photos:

You may visually chronicle your improvement by taking before-and-after pictures of yourself. To ensure that your comparisons are accurate, be careful to utilize the same lighting and positions throughout.

Keep an eye on both your weight and your body composition:

You should weigh yourself on a regular basis, but you should also bear in mind that your weight might change owing to variables such as the retention of water and the building of muscle. If you want a more precise view of your progress, consider employing body composition data like your body fat %.

Monitor your nutrition:

Maintain a food journal or use an app that tracks nutrition to record your meals and snacks. This can assist you in seeing patterns and enabling you to make necessary modifications to your diet.

Track Your Progress Using Fitness Metrics:

You should keep track of metrics pertinent to your fitness goals, such as your running times, the number of push-ups or pull-ups you can complete, and your improvements in flexibility.

Evaluate How You Currently Feel:

Pay attention to how you are feeling on both a mental and a physical level. Significant markers of development include elevated levels of energy, improved mood, and general improvement in well-being.

Create and Evaluate Your Goals:

Create goals that can be easily measured, and make it a habit to evaluate them periodically. You should readjust your objectives as necessary in light of your progress and the shifting emphasis in your life.

A FEW SUGGESTIONS TO HELP YOU SET REALISTIC EXPECTATIONS:

Recognize That Making Progress Will Take Some Time:

Be conscious that significant improvements in one's health and fitness may take time to occur. Remember to be patient and to maintain your dedication throughout the long haul.

Establish Objectives That Can Be Achieved:

Establish objectives that are specific, measurable, and within your reach that correspond to your existing fitness level and lifestyle—separate highly ambitious objectives into a series of smaller, more doable goals.

Put Less Emphasis on the End Result and More on the Process:

Instead of focusing entirely on the result of your efforts to improve your health and fitness, try to take pleasure in the journey itself. Honor even the most insignificant of your achievements as you go.

Be Aware of Setbacks and Plateaus in Your Progress:

Realize that advancement does not always occur in a linear fashion. It is very natural to reach a plateau or experience a setback, and doing so can bring chances for learning and adaptation.

Stay away from comparisons that aren't accurate:

Try not to judge your advancement based on that of others. Each individual's journey is unique, and major differences might arise from variables such as genetics and place of departure.

Pay Attention to Your Body:

Pay heed to the cues that your body gives you. Burnout or injury can result from overtraining or pushing oneself beyond limits. The need for downtime and recovery is integral to the advancement process.

Keep an open mind:

Maintain a flexible attitude toward the achievement of your goals. Life has no guarantees, and your priorities or circumstances might sometimes shift.

Recognize and Honor Accomplishments:

Recognize and honor your accomplishments, no matter how insignificant they may appear, and celebrate them. The use of positive reinforcement may increase motivation.

CHAPTER 9: SAFETY AND INJURY PREVENTION

IMPORTANCE OF SAFETY IN THE GYM

It is of the utmost significance to emphasize safety at the gym to safeguard your physical well-being, provide a productive and pleasurable experience, and maximize your potential for physical improvement. The following is a list of various reasons why ensuring everyone's safety in the fitness center should be a top priority:

1. Preventing Harm to Others:

The primary goal of safety measures is to protect workers from being hurt. If done properly, various workouts and gym equipment might be safe to one's health. Form and technique must be correct at all times in order to reduce the likelihood of damage.

2. Development over the Long Term:

Injuries might derail your fitness development, and you may be required to take some time off from exercising. Achieving long-term fitness objectives requires maintaining a consistent workout routine and avoiding injuries make it possible.

3. Health and Wellness of the Body:

Your physical and mental wellness should always come before anything else. If you disregard safety precautions, you might end up with acute injuries like muscular strains or sprains, as well as chronic problems that may manifest themselves over the course of time.

4. Instilling a Sense of Confidence:

You are more likely to push your boundaries, experiment with new exercises, and establish and accomplish challenging fitness objectives if you believe the gym environment supports and encourages you.

5. Making the Most of the Benefits:

You may maximize the benefits of your workouts by ensuring that appropriate form and safety procedures are always followed. Both efficient and effective training will lead to higher results.

6. Serving as an Example:

Setting a positive example for others, especially novices or folks with less experience who may turn to you for direction, is one of the best things you can do in a fitness facility.

7. The Gym Lifestyle:

A culture of safety helps to promote an environment that is inviting and inclusive in a gym. It encourages members to behave in a manner that is courteous and kind toward one another.

8. Lessening One's Obligation to Pay:

Providing a risk-free atmosphere for patrons is an obligation that fitness centers must fulfill. You may assist in decreasing the danger of accidents as well as the possibility of legal troubles if you adhere to the safety requirements.

Advice to Keep in Mind to Ensure Your Safety at the Gym

1. Acquire the Appropriate Technique:

Spend some time learning the proper form for each exercise you do, and then make sure you practice what you've learned. If you are uncertain, it is best to seek the advice of a fitness specialist.

2. Preparation and decompression:

Always ensure that before you exercise, you warm up your muscles with mild aerobic activity and dynamic stretching and that after your workout, you cool down with some static stretching.

3. Make Use Of Observers:

Utilize a spotter to aid you and safeguard your safety whenever you are lifting large weights, especially while performing exercises such as the bench press or squat.

4. Be Aware of Your Constraints:

Make slow, steady progress and avoid overdoing your weights or executing workouts that are too difficult for your fitness level.

5. Keep yourself hydrated:

During exercise, maintaining adequate water is critical for avoiding overheating as well as cramping in the muscles.

6. Utilize All Necessary Protective Gear

Always ensure you are wearing suitable training clothes and using any essential safety equipment, such as weightlifting belts, gloves, or wrist wraps.

Cleaning the Equipment: It is important to clean the equipment before and after usage to avoid the transmission of germs and keep the area where you exercise clean.

7. Remember That This Is Your Space:

Always keep proper gym etiquette in mind and give other people adequate space so they may work out in a secure environment.

8. Put in a Help Request:

In order to get guidance or clarification on the proper use of equipment or workout forms, you can ask the personnel at the gym or experienced gym-goers for help.

9. Issues to be Reported:

Notify a gym staff member as soon as possible if you discover any broken or faulty equipment, as well as any potential risks to your safety.

GUIDANCE ON INJURY PREVENTION

Injury prevention is an essential component of any exercise regimen. Follow these tips for good warm-up and cool-down routines to lessen the chance of injury and improve your entire workout experience:

Warm-up Procedure

Begin with light cardio:

Warm up for 5-10 minutes with mild aerobic activity such as brisk walking, running in place, or cycling. This boosts your core body temperature and promotes blood flow.

Stretching Dynamically:

After your little cardio, stretch dynamically. Controlled motions are used to improve your range of motion progressively. Leg swings arm, and hip circles are all great dynamic stretches.

Muscles should be activated:

Include activities that will engage the muscles you will use during your workout. For example, perform bodyweight squats or leg lifts if you're planning a leg exercise.

Gradual Development:

The warm-up intensity should gradually increase to prepare your body for the main activity. Begin with low-intensity motions and progressively raise the level of difficulty.

Warm-up Exercises:

Perform one or two sets of the first exercise with lesser weights if you're undertaking resistance training to prepare your muscles and joints further.

Mental Concentration

Use the warm-up to prepare yourself for your workout mentally. Concentrate on your objectives and envision a good training session.

Cool-down Procedure

Gradual Decrease in Intensity:

Reduce the intensity of your workouts progressively toward the finish of your session. Slow down your speed if you've been exercising cardio.

Stretching that is static:

Perform static stretches after your workout to enhance flexibility and alleviate muscular strain. Stretch for 15-30 seconds, focusing on key muscle groups. Stretches for the quadriceps, hamstrings, calves, and chest are some examples.

Deep Inhalation:

Deep breathing techniques will help you calm your body and drop your pulse rate. To relax the nervous system, take slow, deep breaths while stretching.

Nutrition and Hydration:

Replace lost fluids throughout your workout by rehydrating with water or a sports drink. To aid recovery, consume a balanced lunch or snack, including protein and carbs, within an hour of your workout.

Optional foam rolling:

Foam rolling can assist in relieving muscular tension and stiffness. Spend a few minutes focusing on particular areas of tension or discomfort.

Consider and Plan:

Make use of the cool-down phase to reflect on your workout and create goals for your next session. Consider what went well and where you might make improvements.

Rest and recuperation:

Rest and rehabilitation are critical for injury prevention. Ensure you get adequate sleep and give your body time to recover from your workouts.

WHAT TO DO IN CASE OF AN INJURY OR DISCOMFORT

If an injury or discomfort occurs during exercise, it is critical to respond quickly and effectively to avoid further damage and allow a safe and successful recovery process. Here's what you should do:

You should immediately quit the activity when you first discover an injury or discomfort, whether a quick acute pain or a lingering aching. Continuing to exercise despite pain might aggravate the injury and lead to more serious outcomes. Resting at this point is critical to avoiding further strain or harm.

Determine the extent of the injury or suffering. Determine if the problem is mild and may be resolved with rest and self-care or whether it requires more severe treatment. Minor concerns such as muscular strains, minor sprains, or slight soreness from overuse are common. Considerable injuries may cause considerable pain, swelling, loss of function, or obvious deformity.

If you are unclear about the seriousness of the injury or if it is a reoccurring issue, get medical treatment. For a proper examination and diagnosis, see a healthcare expert such as a doctor, physical therapist, or sports medicine specialist. They can give professional advice on the nature of the injury as well as the best course of treatment and rehabilitation.

In certain circumstances, self-care approaches may be sufficient to handle minor injuries or discomfort at home. Here are some general actions to take if you have a small injury:

Rest: Allow your body to recuperate by avoiding activities that aggravate the pain or discomfort. Rest is critical for healing.

To relieve swelling and inflammation, apply ice to the damaged region. Place a cloth or towel between the ice and your skin to avoid frostbite. During the first 48 hours following the injury, apply ice for 15-20 minutes every 1-2 hours.

Use a compression bandage to assist in reducing swelling if necessary. Ensure it's snug but not too tight to avoid cutting off circulation.

Elevation: When feasible, elevate the damaged location above the level of your heart. This can aid in the reduction of edema and the promotion of blood circulation.

Over-the-counter pain medications such as ibuprofen or acetaminophen can help relieve discomfort and decrease inflammation. If you are concerned about drug interactions or allergies, follow the suggested dose guidelines and see a healthcare expert.

Gentle, regulated range-of-motion exercises may be effective throughout the rehabilitation process for some injuries. These should be done under the supervision of a healthcare physician or physical therapist.

Protect and support the damaged region using braces, splints, or crutches, as a healthcare practitioner suggests.

Follow Medical counsel: If you've obtained expert medical counsel, stick to the prescribed treatment plan. Physical therapy activities, rehabilitation, or certain drugs may be included.

Throughout the rehabilitation process, paying attention to your body is critical. Seek medical help immediately if pain or discomfort persists or increases after self-care efforts. Ignoring chronic pain might lead to chronic problems or difficulties.

As you recuperate, gradually reintroduce activities and exercises as your healthcare professional recommends. Resuming your usual training regimen too quickly will raise your chance of re-injury. Focus on gradually and carefully regaining strength, flexibility, and endurance.

CHAPTER 10: BUILDING A SUPPORT SYSTEM

BENEFITS OF HAVING A WORKOUT BUDDY

A workout partner or a support network may make or break your fitness journey. It has several benefits beyond motivation and can considerably improve your general well-being. Whether you're just getting started or have been working out for years, having someone to share your fitness experiences with cannot be understated. This essay will examine the advantages of having a workout companion or a support network.

First and foremost, a workout partner or a support network may incentivize you to stick to your fitness regimen. Let's be honest: there are days when the sofa's appeal outweighs the gym's pull. In such circumstances, knowing that someone is counting on you to show up can be a great motivator to get started. Your exercise companion may be an accountability buddy, ensuring you stick to your fitness plan. This obligation to someone else might help you resist the urge to miss an exercise.

Furthermore, having a workout partner typically makes exercise more fun. Exercise is transformed from a duty into a pleasant activity. You may compete in friendly competition, laugh together, and enjoy great moments. This social factor may convert your training practice from a chore to something you enjoy. It becomes simpler to prioritize fitness in your everyday life when you look forward to your workouts since you'll be spending time with a buddy.

A workout partner can increase your exercise performance and provide encouragement and enjoyment. Having a partner allows for constructive criticism and encouragement. During weightlifting exercises, you may spot each other, guaranteeing appropriate form and lowering the chance of injury. Running or cycling, for example, can help you push your boundaries and accomplish quicker speeds or greater distances than you would on your own.

In addition to the physical benefits, exercising with a buddy or support network can improve your emotional health. Physical exercise produces endorphins, which are natural mood enhancers. This experience can boost sentiments of togetherness and enjoyment when shared with others. Furthermore, social connection can help alleviate feelings of loneliness or isolation, which is especially significant for those who do not have a large social network outside of their workout routines.

Having a workout partner or a support network may also be a great source of motivation and inspiration. As you and your fitness partners work together to reach your objectives, you can see each other's progress and celebrate each other's accomplishments. These shared triumphs may serve as a strong reminder of what is possible, inspiring you to keep pushing yourself. It's motivating to witness someone you know overcome obstacles and progress in their fitness journey because it tells you you can, too.

Working out with others might also help to diversify your exercise regimen. Different people may have different fitness hobbies and levels of skill. You can find new hobbies and widen your fitness horizons by engaging in activities you might not have explored independently. A buddy, for example, may introduce you to yoga, rock climbing, or kickboxing, bringing diversity to your routines and minimizing monotony.

A workout partner may also serve as a safety net for your fitness ambitions. Whether trying out new hobbies or pushing your limits in old ones, having someone keep an eye on you might bring peace of mind. In an emergency or injury, your spouse can aid or seek help. This additional layer of security might help you feel more confident and eager to take on new challenges in your fitness quest.

Aside from a workout companion, a larger support network may provide several benefits in attaining and sustaining your fitness objectives. This network might consist of family members, friends, coworkers, or even online groups of like-minded people. A support network's range of viewpoints and experiences is a significant advantage. You may learn from others' achievements and failures, gain insights into various training approaches, and receive useful nutrition, recovery, and goal-setting guidance.

Your support network can also provide a strong sense of belonging and acceptance. You feel validated and encouraged when you discuss your fitness experience with others who understand and support your goals. This sense of belonging may boost your self-esteem and self-worth, promoting a good body image and a more favorable connection with exercise and diet.

A support network may also update you on the newest fitness trends, research, and best practices. Members of your network may post articles, films, or personal experiences that give useful insights and direction. This knowledge can help you make more educated fitness decisions, leading to greater outcomes and safer practices.

Another benefit of having a support network is the possibility of responsibility and competitiveness. While a workout partner can give instant accountability, a larger network can provide a more comprehensive system of checks and balances. Sharing your efforts and goals with a bigger group helps instill a feeling of accountability to keep your promises. Additionally, friendly rivalry within your network can motivate you to achieve and always improve.

TIPS FOR FINDING A WORKOUT PARTNER

Finding the appropriate workout companion may help you stay motivated accountable, and enjoy your workouts. Here are some pointers to help you locate a workout buddy:

Consult with your friends and family: Begin by contacting friends and family members who may share similar fitness objectives or hobbies. The presence of someone you know and trust might make the collaboration more comfortable.

Use Social Media: Social media platforms, particularly fitness-related ones like Instagram or fitness-focused Facebook groups, may be excellent locations to meet possible exercise partners. You may use hashtags about your fitness hobbies to find them or join online fitness forums.

Fitness applications: Some fitness applications, such as Strava or MyFitnessPal, allow you to connect with other users and find exercise partners. You can look for individuals in your neighborhood with similar fitness objectives or hobbies.

Many gyms have bulletin boards where members may post ads asking for workout companions. Check the bulletin board at your gym or ask the staff if they can help you connect with others.

Fitness Classes: Attending fitness classes at a gym or studio is a great way to meet possible exercise companions. Start talking with your classmates to determine if you are interested in working out together outside class.

Local Sports and Athletic Clubs: Participating in local sports or athletic clubs linked to your hobbies, such as tennis or hiking groups, can be a great way to meet exercise companions who share your enthusiasm for a particular activity.

Meetup.com and Eventbrite frequently feature fitness-related events, group runs, and exercise meetings. These activities might provide an opportunity to meet other people interested in fitness.

Workplace Wellness Programs: Some places of employment provide wellness programs or fitness challenges. If your employer offers such programs, you may be able to locate coworkers who are interested in working out together.

Explore online fitness groups and forums where individuals discuss their fitness adventures, offer suggestions, and seek exercise partners. Bodybuilding.com and Reddit's fitness subreddits are terrific places to start.

Personal Trainers and Group Fitness Instructors: If you work with a personal trainer or attend group fitness courses, your trainer or teacher may be able to link you with other customers or participants interested in teaming up.

Participate in local fitness activities such as charity races, obstacle courses, and fun fitness challenges. Fitness enthusiasts frequently attend these gatherings, hoping to meet people with similar interests.

Choosing a workout partner whose fitness level, goals, and schedule are compatible with yours is critical. A good exercise relationship requires effective communication and clear expectations. Before you commit, talk about your fitness goals, favorite training types, availability, and how you intend to support each other's goals.

POWER OF ACCOUNTABILITY IN STAYING ON TRACK

Accountability is a strong force that may greatly influence your capacity to stick to your objectives, whether connected to health, personal growth, work, or any other element of life. It entails accepting accountability for your actions, decisions, and commitments, and it frequently entails discussing your progress and objectives with people who can hold you responsible. In this essay, we will look at responsibility's powerful role in assisting individuals to reach their goals and stay on track.

1. Commitment and accountability:

Accountability is really about making a commitment to yourself and accepting responsibility for your actions. When you make a goal and hold yourself accountable, you are more likely to take it seriously and prioritize it. The core of accountability's strength is this dedication and sense of duty.

2. Clarity and Focus on Goals:

Accountability assists you in properly defining and staying focused on your goals. When you know you'll be reporting your progress to others, you're more likely to create specified, measurable, attainable, relevant, and time-bound (SMART) goals. This clarity allows you to track your progress and make required changes.

3. Persistence and Motivation:

One of the major advantages of accountability is its capacity to increase motivation and consistency. Knowing that someone is keeping track of your progress or that you have committed to someone else may be quite motivating. It motivates you to persevere in your work even when faced with hurdles or diversions.

4. Dealing with Procrastination:

Procrastination is a typical impediment to goal achievement. You have a built-in method to prevent procrastination when you are held accountable. The fact that you'll have to report your progress might be a significant barrier to procrastination.

5. Enhanced Productivity:

Accountability can lead to higher productivity since it forces you to manage your time better. You become more conscious of how you spend your time and attempt to prioritize things relevant to your goals.

6. Adaptation and Problem Solving:

When held accountable, you are more willing to confront problems and barriers. Instead of giving up, you become a problem solver, discovering solutions to overcome obstacles. Accountability promotes flexibility and resilience.

7. Positive Peer Influence:

Being responsible to someone else sometimes entails seeking assistance from peers or mentors. This support network may create positive peer pressure, where the dedication and development of individuals around you impact you. It motivates you to increase your standards and provide your best effort.

8. Motivation and Celebration:

Accountability partners or groups may support you and share your accomplishments with you. Recognizing your accomplishments, no matter how minor builds your confidence and strengthens your dedication to your goals.

Personal Development and Growth:

Personal growth and development can be facilitated through accountability. It promotes self-reflection and self-development by assessing your progress and identifying growth opportunities.

10. Improved Relationships:

Accountability frequently entails cultivating relationships with those who share your aims or values. These partnerships can help you enhance your social ties while giving you a sense of belonging and support.

11. Measurable Results:

Accountability provides a clear means to track your progress. Regular check-ins, reports, or milestones allow you to evaluate your progress and make data-driven decisions about your future moves.

12. Reduced Risk of Relapse:

When faced with setbacks or problems, accountability can assist in preventing backsliding or falling off the wagon. Knowing you have a support structure reduces the likelihood of quitting your ambitions after encountering setbacks.

13. Better Time Management:

Accountability promotes improved time management and work prioritization. You become more efficient in your everyday routines, ensuring that you constantly designate time to focus on your goals.

14. Improved Self-Discipline:

Accountability promotes self-discipline by instilling the habit of following through on promises and focusing on your goals.

15. Habits for Longevity:

Accountability assists you in developing and maintaining long-term behaviors that lead to success. Rather than seeking short cures, you are urged to make long-term adjustments in your behavior and lifestyle.

16. Trusted and respected:

Accountability gains the respect and trust of others. When you constantly keep your promises, you build a reputation as someone dependable.

17. Loop of Positive Feedback:

Accountability establishes a positive feedback loop. As you grow and achieve, it strengthens your dedication to your goals and pushes you to strive for even greater accomplishment.

18. Improved Decision-Making:

Accountability promotes deliberate decision-making. You become more aware of your decisions and how they relate to your objectives.

19.-Increased Self-Awareness:

Accountability allows you to understand yourself better, your capabilities, and your areas for growth. This self-awareness may be a benefit in both personal and professional development.

20. Achieving Lofty Objectives:

The potential of accountability to urge you toward ambitious goals is its most significant strength. You may pursue and achieve goals that may have appeared intimidating or unreachable on your own with the support and structure given by accountability.

CONCLUSION

In conclusion, starting your fitness adventure with "The Beginner's Guide to Starting Gym Workouts" is an important step toward a better and more satisfying life. We've covered the fundamentals of gym exercises in this booklet, from setting clear objectives to building a well-rounded exercise regimen to comprehending good form and nutrition.

Remember that every fitness journey is different, and improvement is not necessarily linear. Continue to be patient, driven, and, most importantly, consistent. The gym is more than simply a place to grow muscle; it's also a place to develop resilience, discipline, and self-confidence. You will not only observe physical alterations as you traverse the difficulties and successes of your exercises, but you will also experience the wonderful mental and emotional advantages that fitness provides.

Your increased knowledge and commitment will pave the path for a healthier, happier, and more energetic future. So, confidently enter that gym, and let your path to a better you begin. With each rep, set, and session, embrace the sweat, taste the growth, and cherish the sense of success. The road to a healthier, more vibrant you begin here, and with dedication and commitment, the sky is the limit. So throw on your sneakers, grab a water bottle, and begin this fantastic adventure to a better and happier self. Your future self will be grateful!